Best Breville Juicer Juicing Recipes: Healthy And Delicious

How To Make Unique Breville Juicer Juices New For 2013

By: Stacey Turner

978-1482376593

1482376598

TABLE OF CONTENTS

CONTENTS

Stacey Turner

DEDICATION

This book is dedicated to Emily and Steve as they were influential in helping to get this book put together.

Chapter 1- Benefits Of Juicing

The advantages of juicing have been documented over the years and are quite numerous. Quite a number of countries including the USA currently have quite a number of obese persons. the prevalence of certain ailments are also on the increase including cancer, diabetes and heart disease as there is an increase in the consumption of sugar and fat filled processed and fast foods.

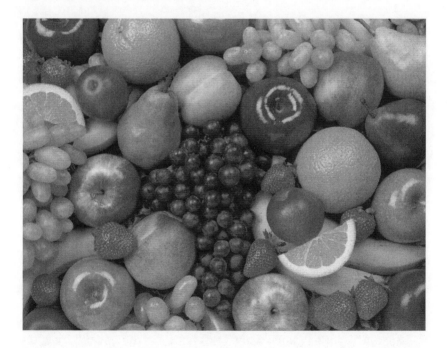

In the last number of years a new trend has come to the fore, which is the increased interest in healthy and organic foods. It appears that more and more individuals are coming to the realization that the way that they eat has an effect on how long they live.

It is not only health professionals and athletes that are starting to discover that juicing can assist them to have a longer life span as it is a much healthier option in the long run.

Advantages

Doing juicing for health reasons provides essential minerals, vitamins, antioxidants and nutrients for the bodies to grow and regenerate cells, have a stronger immune system and help with repair.

One of the major benefits of juicing is getting the nutritional benefits of raw foods. Fiber can be found in copious amounts in many fruits and vegetables and the benefit of this gets lost when the fiber does not get unlocked in the digestive system. The process of juicing releases the nutrition of the fiber so one can accrue the full benefits.

We typically do not eat the pits, seeds and peelings of vegetables. These parts are filled with essential nutrients and they are typically discarded. A high quality juicer will extract the juice from the entire fruit or vegetable including the seeds, pits and peelings so all the minerals and vitamins would not be lost.

Enzymes are killed by heat. A great juicer will not emit a lot of heat so the enzymes will be preserved.

Using a great juicer will reducing the amount of foaming. This foam represents oxidation and when this occurs the benefit of the antioxidant will be lower. The less the foam is, the more benefits you will get from antioxidants.

Juice is a great meal or snack replacement that satiates hunger. A lot of dieters state that the juices help them to shed the excess weight without the cravings.

The antioxidants that are present in the juices will help to detoxify the body and also assist with the elimination of toxins, chemicals, preservatives and fats that a diet comprised of processed foods tends to leave in the body.

The other benefits of juicing include uplift in mood and more energy. As the body gets cleaned out and detoxified it will be easier to use and access sustaining and restorative nutrients that will improve the way that you feel in the long run. You will be in much better spirits when you have more energy.

Juice is one of the foods that easy to absorb and digest especially in a concentrated form. The process of juicing makes things easier to digest and the body gets the necessary benefits from food.

Preparing your own juice will allow you to prepare any combination of vegetables or fruits that you want and the great thing is that you will really know what the ingredients are.

There are no real disadvantages that can be made mention of. In short juicing is beneficial for you.

The advantages of juicing start with begin with the creation of your own mixes of drinks and it has a healthy end result as it helps to fight diseases. Along with that there are also the benefits of getting more nutrition for the body for the growth and healing by making the nutrients in fiber readily available

Juicing provides more than one way to get the most nutrition from the food that you eat. Apart from that, juicing uses all parts of fruits and vegetables which results in a maximization of nutrients.

As a result of this juicing is a great way to get the majority of the nutrients that can be found in vegetables and fruits. As soon as you get used to juicing and start to see the benefits of juicing like the increase in energy, there will be no reason to stop.

Drinking fruit and vegetable juice that is freshly prepared can be done by any individual that has an interest in improving their health and be better able to resist disease and illness and delay the onset of aging while boosting vitality and energy. These vegetables and fruits are filled with antioxidants, phytochemicals and enzymes and other things that help to promote good health.

Major Advantages of Juicing

The Advantages of Juicing- Why Juice?

Advantages of juicing- remember that the advantages cannot be overlooked. As individuals try to find healthier ways to live and healthier options to eat, juicing has become increasingly popular.

It does not only provide you with a wide range of minerals, vitamins and nutrients but there is also fiber, antioxidants and enzymes. All over the world there are persons who will include a glass of fresh vegetable or fruit juice in their diet. Outlined below is more information on the benefits of juicing.

Juicing Aids with Digestion

Stacey Turner

One of the great benefits if juicing is that it assists the digestive system in the body to work more effectively. It helps to alleviate constipation and also lowers the threat of colon cancer. It also cleanses and detoxifies. The absorption of the juice from fresh vegetable and fruits is much easier than when whole foods are consumed.

Nutritional Advantages

Many individuals are aware that the nutritional value is the greatest benefit of juicing raw vegetables and fruits. These foods are filled with minerals and vitamins in addition to other vital substances that are required. These antioxidants and enzymes help the body to resist the onset of certain diseases.

Alleviate the Symptoms of Numerous Diseases

A lot of individuals will find these benefits of juicing surprising. For instance the pain of arthritis can be relieved with ginger juice. Joint pain that is the result of gout can be eased with fresh cherry juice and constipation can be relieved with fresh carrot juice. There are a number of ways that fresh vegetable and fruit juice can make you feel great.

Tips for Juicing

Oxidation tends to take place quickly in juice. When this occurs, the amount of nutrients in the juice begins to diminish. This is why it is essential to consume the juice as soon as you can after you prepare it. A number of juicers are better at slowing down the process of oxidation than others and will allow you to be able to make enough juice to last a couple of days. Just remember that the quicker you drink it, the more nutrition you will get from it.

You will able to use the juicer to create some great recipes. You can mix the vegetables and fruits to get the most nutrition or just select one. Quite a number of recipes can be found online but when you purchase a juicer, it will come with a recipe book as well. never be afraid to experiment, you might just create a great tasting, nutritious drink.

The benefits of juicing are much more than taste and convenience. This is the essential part of a lifestyle that is healthy and you will be amazed by the boost in energy that you get. A lot of individuals attribute their long life to juicing in addition to their youthful look. You will realize that after just a few days of juicing that the skin will appear to be younger and brighter looking and that you will have greater vitality and lots more energy. There is no need to delay the process to start enjoying the benefits of juicing.

Choosing the right juicer to suit your needs can be a bit difficult. The question is whether or not a twin gear (triturating) juicer, masticating juicer or centrifugal juicer is right for you? You may wonder which juicer will extract the juice from wheatgrass or spinach. There may even be the question of which juicer is able to make ice cream and nut butters as well.

One of the most popular lines of juicers on the market today is the Breville juicer. One of the reasons for this is that it comes with quite a number of great features. For instance one of the major benefits of the Breville juicer is that it will never get stuck or slow down no matter what it is that is being juiced. The thing that enables all of this is the RPM speed and the motor that the machines have.

The juicers are extremely easy to use. They only have to be turned on and the vegetables and fruits fed into it with the use of a plunger which comes with the machine. The juicers also come equipped with a brush that facilitates quick and easy clean up. If it is a high quality juicer that you are looking for then the Breville juicer is the one to select.

The company originated in Australia and has branches in the United Kingdom and the United States. The company is renowned for manufacturing great kitchen appliances like grills, espresso machines, toast makers and fruit juicers which all sport a great design and function exceptionally making it one of the most popular brands on the market.

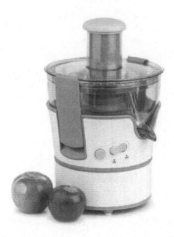

Major Features and Advantages of the Breville Juicers

The Breville juicers are centrifugal machines that come with a number of advantages. The advantages of the juicers are outlined below:

Best Breville Juicing Recipes

It comes with a 600 to 1000 watts output with a three quarter horsepower motor that enables the quick juicing of the hardiest of vegetables in addition to being a durable machine that can be used to juice multiple times per day.

High juice yield can be acquired as a result of the motor which has revolutions of 13000 to 14500 per minute. In essence a quart of juice can be produced every minute. One has to watch the pitcher carefully as it will fill up pretty quickly.

The Breville juicer is extremely easy to put together and take apart making cleaning a simple process. The juicer can be placed in a dishwasher, all that you have to do is to use the brush that comes with it to clean the blade and wire mesh beforehand.

One of the models of the Breville juice extractor, the Juice Fountain comes with a three inch chute which enables the user top place whole vegetables and fruits in the machine, or they can just be cut up in large chunks, saving on time.

The juicers not only work effectively but come with a great design that fist into the contemporary kitchen.

This brand sports a number of juice extractors which permit the selection of a model that best suits the budget and juicing needs.

The juicers are priced reasonably though they come with a lot of great features that many of the other juicers that cost more do not have.

CHAPTER 2- GETTING STARTED WITH JUICING

A lot of individuals that start to juice notice that they have more energy and stamina.

The detoxifying and cleansing effect of the fresh juices also helps to build up that strength. Anytime the body is not filled with toxins it happens to work much better and has more energy. Drinking fresh juices does might help to improve the way the kidneys and liver function. These are two major organs that help with the detox and elimination process

Fresh juices are filled with Magnesium, Potassium and B complex vitamins which are all critical in helping to maintain the regular energy levels.

To improve energy, begin by having the juice recipes that include spinach, parsley and carrot, which are all filled with the nutrients that are necessary for energy. Always have a container of juice tucked away in the refrigerator that you can have throughout the course of the day. In a few days you will start to see the difference.

Flu and Colds

Adults tend to have at least three to four colds each winter and those that spend time with the smaller children tend to have it even more. A lot of personal plans get disrupted and school and work gets missed.

There are a few things that you can do to lower the chances of getting a flu or cold, or simply just decrease the duration and severity.

Internal Protection

A reduction in the level of effectiveness of the immune system is the main factor in getting a cold. In a world that is filled with bacteria and viruses, having good resistance and remaining healthy is not a fluke. The immune system has to be strong. You have to view the immune system as an internal security force that is always monitoring the activities in the body and looking for any sign of flu and cold viruses.

Research has indicated that a few nutrients can have a great effect on the immune system by boosting it so that it can effectively deal with the viruses.

Juicing consistently, particularly in the months that flu and cold is prevalent will boost the function of the immune system. Fresh fruit and vegetable juices fill the body with the necessary nutrients that have been shown to be vital in the way the immune system responds. These include B complex Vitamins, Zinc, Beta-Carotene and Vitamin C.

Vitamin C appears to be vital in practically every function of the immune system. Many studies have indicated that Vitamin C boosts the immune system in a number of ways. It augments the production of antibodies that prevents infections from spreading. Citrus juices like lemon, orange and grapefruit are filled with Vitamin C. a regular sized orange is filled with the recommended daily dose of Vitamin C.

Beta Carotene is a great immune system booster as it can be converted to Vitamin A as is necessary. It helps to maintain the mucous the membranes and reduces the instances of infections as it builds up the defense mechanisms of the body. Green juices like cabbage, kale, beet greens and spinach are filled with Beta Carotene. This can be found in copious amounts in apples and carrots.

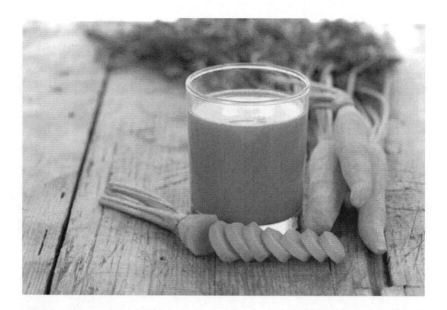

Juicing for Weight Loss

Despite what many people may think there is no great secret to weight loss. It is basically require the consumption of fewer calories on a daily basis. Any weight loss program that is properly prepared will have individuals consuming between 1200 to 1500 calories on a daily basis.

Statistics indicate that approximately 84 percent of adults in the United States that are older than twenty years of age tend to be overweight. This is due to the consumption of the standard American diet which is filled with salt, saturated fats and calories and is low in minerals and vitamins. This, along with a lifestyle that is sedentary contributes to the weight problems.

Juicing is a great way to lower the consumption of calories while supplying the necessary minerals and vitamins that are required to sustain energy. it is great to help lower the pangs of hunger that tend to occur with programs geared toward weight loss.

Anytime you opt to juice something you will automatically be reducing the consumption of high cholesterol and fat in the diet. Attempt to use juice as a replacement meal for one or two meals per day. Always consume one meal every day that is balanced. It should consist of fiber in the form of vegetables, salad with a dressing that is low in calories and a small portion of protein.

Recipes for juicing with parsley or carrot also help to reduce those cravings and curtail the appetite. They also help to maintain the correct levels of blood sugar cutting down on the fluctuations that can occur in blood sugar when one is one a program geared toward weight loss.

Try apple and grapefruit in the mornings. As the fruit juice has more calories than the vegetable juices they can be diluted to help lower the number of calories that are consumed. For instance, one can have a nice green drink for lunch made with spinach, parsley and carrot.

Getting the right amount of exercise is another essential way to lose weight. All that you have to do is have fifteen to twenty minutes of exercise daily along with the juicing to maximize on the positive results. A nice walk every day can help burn calories.

Cleansing the Liver with Juicing

The juicer is the best kitchen appliance that can help to maintain the health of the organs, the liver in particular.

The liver is the biggest gland that we have and is the only organ which can renew itself even if some of it sustains damage.

One of the major functions of the liver is to act as a detoxifier for the body. It works to get rid of the harmful substances before that can get into the bloodstream. The effects of drugs and alcohol are neutralized by the liver.

Juicing can be used to clean the liver occasionally and can play a vital role in the maintenance of good health. Juices that are fresh lower the pressure that is placed on the liver and gives it the opportunity to recover. While the liver is being cleansed it will be cleansed of the built up toxins and work much more efficiently in the long run.

All the green juices can help the liver to detox particularly those with cucumbers, dandelion leaves, kale, zucchini, parsley and spinach. Always put some carrots in the green juice as it can end up being too strong and can affect the throat. A great way to cleanse the liver is to have some beetroot juice so try some recipes that includes beets and apples. Having grapefruit and lemon in the morning can also help with the detox of the liver.

Putting the Juice Program Together

When you start to juice, it is best to put together a juicing program that is best suited for one's health goals and specific lifestyle. Start by having a glass of juice on the morning and after a period of time you will start to experience the positive effects including better regularity, improved immune function and increased stamina and vitality.

Also have some juice in the afternoon and later on in the day as a natural boost. Think about carrying some juice to work or when you run errands.

It is best to start with carrots. It is the best vegetable juice and is filled with potassium, calcium and a number of trace minerals as well as Vitamins K, E, D, C, B and Beta Carotene. This juice helps to regulate elimination, detox the liver and increase alkalinity to balance the pH of the body. It blends well with other vegetables and a number of fruits like apple.

After that, start by using other fruits and vegetables for juicing. You will get a great head start with the recipes that come with the juicer. There are a lot of great options out there that are extremely tasty.

Bear in mind that fruit and vegetable don't generally mix. There are some exceptions however and those are outlined in the other chapters. As long as you stick to the guidelines you will not make any mistakes.

Tips on Juicing

Of course, everything in life comes with some advice. Any tips that you get on juicing are priceless. That is something that many learn as they get into the process of juicing.

Consume the juices as quickly as possible after juicing as the nutritional value starts to diminish over time. In addition to that as oxidation takes place, the color will change. This does not mean that if is spoilt but many won't want to taste it when the color is off. It is advised to have the juice in twenty four hours but it can be kept for as long as two days. Just remember that there are no preservatives in fresh juice.

You can start by preparing the ingredients for the juice ahead of time. Things go much more quickly if the vegetables/fruits are prepared ahead of time. Everything can be cut up and washed and placed in a container and stored in the refrigerator until it is needed. There really is no excuse not to juice.

N.B.: Bear in mind that nutrients tend to diminish when you start to cut the vegetables up. It does work better to cut those up right before starting to juice. If you are short on time the prepping beforehand is essential.

Making use of the pulp is also a great way to get additional nutrition and save money. This is one tip that I wish I had been aware of when I started juicing as I used to get rid of the pulp until someone made me the wiser. It is pretty easy to use the pulp and it does feel great not to be wasting so much.

The next great juicing tip is store the juice in a glass container. This is something that I learned after doing the wrong thing. I was having carrot juice and decided to carry some to work. I put the juice I required in a plastic container, carried it to work and forgot it on my desk. Suffice it to say that the bottle exploded and my desk had its fill of carrot juice. This would not have occurred if the juice was placed in a glass container. The main point is that it is not prudent to store the juice in plastic. It is best to recycle and use a glass container that you have thrown away otherwise. Also store the juice in the refrigerator if it will not be consumed right away. If the bottle that you are storing it in is not dark you can wrap the bottle with some foil and slow down the process of oxidation.

Also remember that not all vegetables and fruits can be combined or even work well for juicing. The fruits that tend to be mushy like bananas are not great for juicing but can make a great ice cream treat when a blank plate or homogenizer is used in the juicer. Berries do tend to be mushy as well and will not yield a lot of juice unlike oranges or apples.

When too many vegetables and fruits are used it can lead to a juice that has a strange taste. The juices that you purchase in the supermarket that have in lots of produce also have flavoring added to make it taste better. This option does not come with fresh juice so one has to be careful with the combinations. For starts you can use a maximum of three vegetables or fruits and through experimentation come up with other great tasting combinations.

Another great tip is to add some ice cubes to the juice. This will help keep the juice cool and refreshing especially in the summer.

Last but by no means least include a bit of banana in the juice and blend it so that it has a consistency that is like a milkshake. This will soften the taste of the drink and also cut down on the bitter taste that some juices will have like grapefruit.

Chapter 3- Vegetable Juicer Recipes

Everyone loves fresh fruit juice, but the recipes for juicing vegetables can be a bit interesting particularly for the individuals that are just starting out on a raw food diet. Bear in mind that most vegetables are not sweet while fresh fruits are. The question is if there exists some method to have a healthy vegetable juice have a great taste. Of course there is. Some tips are outlined below to help with the preparation of vegetable juices.

Add some carrots or fruits to sweeten the greens and to make it taste a bit better. Individuals that are on a raw food diet or those that love juicing will not only feed unpeeled carrots through the juicer but they will also put in some vegetables like celery and cucumbers. If you want the drink to be sweeter, include some pears or apples. This will not only bump up the flavor but also increase the amount of minerals and vitamins in the vegetable juice.

Opt for organic fresh vegetables. If you are able to, select organic, fresh fruits and vegetables to make great vegetable juice recipes. When the products are fresh they the juice will not only taste better but have more nutritional value as well. Organic products also do were not grown with any chemicals and will better meet your health goals.

When juicing it is advised it is best to keep the skin on the fruits and vegetables which is where most of the nutrients are contained. The Breville juicer will be able to break it all down and extract the essential nutrients that you need.

Purchase a great juicer to get the full benefits of juicing vegetables. A great option is to get one that has a motor of at least 450 watts. The aim is to get the most juice from the vegetables and fruits that you are able to, and retain the strength of the product. it is a fact that some juicers will juice better than others but can prove challenging to clean, so do a bit of research to find the best one that will work for you. It is also better to juice daily with a not so great juicer as opposed to once per week with a fabulous juicer. In spite of this remember to do the necessary research, look at all the relevant reviews and listen to the experts.

Change up the ingredients- use your creativity when it comes to making your vegetable juices for the nutritional value and the taste. Use that imagination and with time work on having more green juices as those are filled with nutrition, can help balance the alkaline in the body and have low sugar content.

Of course there is no set rule for juicing vegetables. You are able to try various vegetable and fruit mixes and become more accustomed to the various tastes. Below are a couple of basic recipes that you can start with.

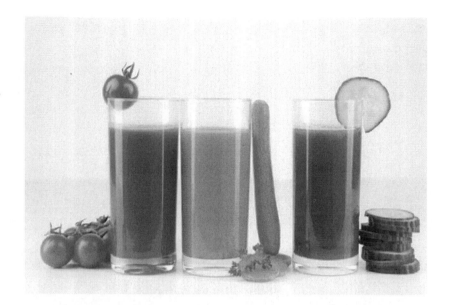

Juicing Recipes

Greens

Ingredients

Handful of grapes

2 big carrots

2 apples

4 stalks kale

2 celery stalks

2 handfuls spinach

Best Breville Juicing Recipes

Preparation

Juice and serve

Pineapple Burst

Ingredients

½ a cucumber

10 strawberries

½ a fresh pineapple

1 large handful fresh baby spinach

Preparation

Juice then pour over ice and enjoy!

Purple-Blast!

Ingredients

Pomegranate

Pineapple

Black or red grapes

Purple cabbage

Preparation

Stacey Turner

Juice and serve

Strawberry Medley

Ingredients

8 Strawberries

2 Carrots

2 Apples

Preparation

Juice and serve

Green Punch

Ingredients

1 green apple

2 cucumbers

2 cups spinach

3 stalks celery

Preparation

Juice and serve

Weight Loss Mix

Best Breville Juicing Recipes

This juice is quick and easy to prepare and makes a great breakfast meal which helps to shed the pounds.

Ingredients

Cucumber

Carrot

Cabbage

Preparation

Juice and serve

Late Breakfast

Ingredients

1 inch ginger

1 apple

1 orange peeled

½ red pepper (sweet)

2 carrots

1 cup red cabbage

1 beet

Stacey Turner

Preparation

Juice and serve

Sweet Potato, Carrot, Ginger & Orange Medley

Ingredients

1 chunk of ginger (bout an inch)

2 ½ sweet potatoes

2-3 skinny carrots

1 regular orange

Preparation

Juice and blend with ice than serve

Vegetable Burst

Ingredients

1" of ginger root

2" turmeric root (powdered turmeric can be added to the juice)

Small tomato

Some basil leaves

½ bunch of kale

Best Breville Juicing Recipes

½ bunch of cilantro

3" chunk of Daikon radish

3 stalks of celery

1 apple (cored)

1 bell pepper

1 very large carrot

1 beet

Preparation

Juice, then run pulp through the juicer once more and serve.

Lemon, Cabbage & Celery

Ingredients

1 lemon

½ head purple cabbage

¾ bunch celery

Preparation

Juice and serve. Really great for cleansing and breaking a fast; the celery juice is filled with minerals that help the kidneys and the lemon and cabbage are great cleansers.

Stacey Turner

Green Fasting Juice

Ingredients

½ a lemon

A few sprigs of flat leaf parsley or cilantro

½ bunch of spinach

1 small cucumber

3" chunk of Daikon radish

½ bunch of kale

4 stalks of celery

Preparation

Juice and serve. It works great when fasting and has wonderful health benefits, if the juice has too strong taste you can dilute it with water. A pear or apple can be used to sweeten it up a bit.

Detox Juice

Ingredients

½ a lemon

1 small apple

1 beet

1 small cucumber

4 celery stalks

5 carrots

Preparation

The juice gives the digestive system a break and lets the body heal. This juice also provides nourishment for the liver and kidney and helps clean them.

Juice then serve

Lemon, Kale & Celery

Ingredients

1 Lemon

1 bunch Kale

1 bunch celery

Preparation

Juice and serve

This juice helps reduce the cravings for salt.

Fennel with Green Juice

Ingredients

Stacey Turner

1 apple

1 lemon

1 bunch celery

1 head lettuce

1 bunch kale

1 fennel bulb with tops

Preparation

Juice and serve

This can serve as a replacement for a meal occasionally for dinner or whenever you want it. It is filled with nutrients and will not cause drowsiness.

Ginger Twist

Ingredients

Small piece of ginger

1 apple

6 carrots

Preparation

Juice and serve

This is a sweet juice that should be had in small amounts. It works well for kids and helps them to get used to drinking natural juices.

Three Green Juice

Ingredients

1 bunch spinach

8 stalks of celery

1 cucumber

Juice all ingredients and enjoy.

Morning Burst

Ingredients

2 Celery Stalks (Optional)

1 Granny Smith Apple

1peeled Kiwi (not too soft)

3 Leaves of Curly Kale

Handful of Parsley

Preparation

Juice starting with the parsley and serve

Stacey Turner

Beet Special

Ingredients

½ lemon-peeled

⅓ pineapple-peeled

1 red grapefruit-peeled

3 large carrots

1 large handful of spinach

1 beet plus greens

Preparation

Juice and serve

Green Treat

Ingredients

Apple

Parsley

Cucumber

Celery

Preparation

Best Breville Juicing Recipes

Juice then serve

Pear & Cucumber Juice

Ingredients

1 cup sugar snap peas

½ large lemon

½ leaf chard

1 cup kale

2 cups spinach

1 peeled cucumber

3 pears

Preparation

Juice and serve

Carrot & Orange Juice

Ingredients

3 oranges (large)

6 carrots

Preparation

Stacey Turner

Juice then serve

Mucus Buster

Ingredients

2 peeled grapefruits

2 Plums (take out seeds)

½ Pineapple

Preparation

Juice then serve

Sweet Beets

Ingredients

Handful of blue berries

1 kiwi

1 beet

1 pear

2 apples

Preparation

Juice then serve

Veggie and Fruit Medley

Ingredients

V8 splash

Carrots

Strawberries

Raspberries

Blueberries

Mango

Preparation

Juice then serve

Mineralizer with a Punch

Ingredients

1 bunch of kale

1 beet (bulb and greens)

¼ inch of ginger

1 lemon

1 apple

Stacey Turner

2 stalks celery

½ a cucumber

4 carrots

Preparation

Juice then serve

Very Berry Mix

Ingredients

2 carrots

2 honey crisp apples or other apple that is sweet

1 cup large red grapes with seeds

½ cup raspberries

1 cup cranberries

1 large beet

Preparation

Juice then serve

Pizza in a Glass

Ingredients

Best Breville Juicing Recipes

1 jalapeno pepper

½ handful of fresh parsley

1 handful of spinach

1 handful of turnip greens

3 garlic cloves

1 onion

5 Roma tomatoes

Preparation

Juice ingredients above then add any of the ingredients below:

1 pinch of sea salt or 1 squirt of Bragg's aminoes

1 tsp of Bragg's apple cider vinegar

1 tbsp olive oil (extra virgin)

Simply Red

Ingredients

1 parsnip

1 celery stalk

1 lemon

Stacey Turner

1 stalk collard green

1 beet

Preparation

Juice then serve

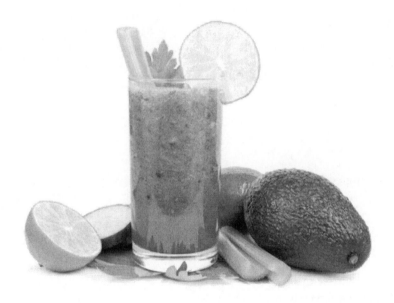

Fabulous Fruit Mix

Ingredients

Radish

2 carrots

1 bunch celery

Best Breville Juicing Recipes

2 bunches of kale

1 cucumber

12 strawberries

2 handfuls of blueberries

3 handfuls of grapes

3 pears

3 apples

2 oranges

2 inches fresh ginger

Preparation

Juice then serve

Easy Breakfast Juice

Ingredients

Strawberries

Pineapple

Apples

Peppers

Stacey Turner

Ginger

Broccoli

Baby Arugula

Kale

Cucumber

Lettuce

Carrots

Celery

Preparation

Juice then serve

Apple & Kale Juice

Ingredients

4-6 stalks kale (based on size of apples)

2 medium apples (jazz or other variety)

Preparation

Juice then serve

Vitamin Filled Juice

Best Breville Juicing Recipes

Ingredients

2 whole long carrots

1 stalk of celery

2 small Fuji apples

¼ of a pineapple

Preparation

Juice then serve

Sweet Greens

Ingredients

5 stalks celery

1 pear

2 handful spinach

1 apple

7 stalks kale

Juice spinach & kale between fruits

Preparation

Juice then serve

CHAPTER 4- FRUIT JUICE RECIPES

Berry Splash

Ingredients

1 apple

1½ cups raspberries

2 cups blueberries

2 cups strawberries

Preparation

Start by coring the apple then juice the raspberries, apple, blueberries and strawberries and serve.

They will be a bit mushy and will not provide a lot of juice but do taste great.

Cucumber and Apple

Ingredients

½ Cucumber

5 Apples

Preparation

Best Breville Juicing Recipes

Core apples then juice the cucumber and apples and serve.

Apple Berry

Ingredients

1 apple

1 cup of blueberries

⅓ cup of strawberries

Preparation

Core the apple then juice the apple, blueberries and strawberries then serve. This drink is filled with antioxidants that fight against aging.

Pear & Kiwi

Ingredients

1 apple

3 pears

2 kiwis

Preparation

Peel kiwis then core apple and pear then juice and serve. It is a great drink for dessert and is pretty sweet.

Apple-Cranberry

Stacey Turner

Ingredients

2 apples

3 carrots

¾ cup cranberries

Preparation

Core apples then juice cranberries, apples and carrots and serve at once. Cranberry is great for the bladder and liver.

Cranberry Pineapple

Ingredients

1 apple

½ cup of cranberries

½ pineapple

Preparation

Core the pineapple and apple. Take the rind off the pineapple then juice the apple, pineapple and cranberries then serve. It has a sweet tangy taste.

Carrot, Orange Juice

Ingredients

4 oranges

1 carrot

½ a melon

Preparation

Peel oranges then take the rind off the melon. Juice oranges, melon and carrots together then serve at once.

Watermelon & Apple

Ingredients

3 slices of watermelon

2 apples

Preparation

Core apples then get rind off watermelon. Juice and serve.

Orange Juice, Strawberries & Grape

Ingredients

1 Orange

1 cup of Grapes (red)

1 cup of Strawberries

Preparation

Peel orange then juice orange, grapes and strawberries and serve. For a great taste juice the grapes and strawberries first then pour that in the glass. Juice the orange and pour it on top for a unique look. This can be done with any juice but place the heavier juices at the bottom.

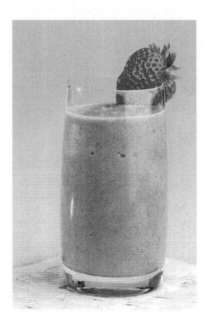

Apricot & Peach

Ingredients

½ cup green grapes

2 apricots

2 peaches

Best Breville Juicing Recipes

Preparation

Take the pits out of the peaches and apricots. Juice the green grapes, apricots and peaches then serve. Makes a great sweet treat!

Orange, Pineapple & Strawberry

Ingredients

1 orange

2-3 slices cored pineapple or ¼ of a pineapple

6-7 strawberries

Preparation

Peel the orange then juice it along with the strawberries and pineapple. Serve at once.

Pomegranate - Apple

Ingredients

2 apples

1 pomegranate (separate seeds from pith)

Preparation

Core apples then separate the arils of the pomegranate. Juice and serve. Makes a great antioxidant punch!

Stacey Turner

Orange Juice

Ingredients

5 peeled oranges

Preparation

It is okay to leave the pith. The oranges can be cut in half to make it easier to feed through the juicer. Use a knife to cut the skin off beforehand.

Orange & Grapefruit

Ingredients

2 oranges

1 grapefruit

Preparation

Peel the orange and grapefruit then cut fruits into sections and juice. For that extra zing a lemon can be added.

Orange with Lemon

Ingredients

1 lemon

3 oranges

Preparation

Peel oranges then juice along with lemon and serve. Be careful not to add too much lemon as it can become bitter to the taste.

Lemonade

Ingredients

¾ cups of agave syrup or honey (easier to mix and lighter- works better than sugar)

6 cups of water

5 whole lemons

Preparation

Cur of or peel lemons then juice them. Pour juice in pitcher with water and add the agave syrup or honey and mix. A few drops of stevia can make the lemonade less bitter.

Apple, Lime & Lemon

Ingredients

2 apples

1 peeled lime

2 lemons

Preparation

Stacey Turner

Core apples and peel lime then juice lime, apple and lemons and serve.

Citrus Pineapple

Ingredients

1 lime

2 oranges

½ a cored Pineapple (remove rind)

Preparation

Peel oranges and lime then juice pineapple, lime and oranges then serve.

ABOUT THE AUTHOR

Stacey Turner is extremely interested in various types of diets and the impact that they really have on any individual that tries them. She is also interested in the impact that these diets have on improving the health of individuals. As a result of this interest she has written a lot of books on various diets from the macrobiotic to the pregnancy diet and so on.

She always had a problem maintaining her weight and was also prone to certain illnesses as a child and a part of her research was geared at finding a solution for her own problem. as she did research she found more and more options and decided to share what she was learning through her books as she was well aware that there were others like her out there trying to find the right solution for their problems.

Stacey is not trying to convince anyone that one diet is better than the next, she opts instead to present all the facts and leave the reader to make the final decision at the end of it all whether or not they will opt to fully try a diet or simply modify what they currently eat to include some of the options.